how my body works

moving

Joan Gowenlock

Wayland

how my body works

Breathing
Eating
Growing
Moving
Sleeping
Staying Healthy

Editor: Anna Girling
Designer: Jean Wheeler

First published in 1992 by
Wayland (Publishers) Ltd
61 Western Road, Hove
East Sussex BN3 1JD, England

British Library Cataloguing in Publication Data
Gowenlock, Joan
Moving.—(How my body works)
I. Title   II. Series
531.11

ISBN 0 7502 0360 9

Typeset by Dorchester Typesetting Group Ltd
Printed and bound in Belgium by Casterman S.A.

All words printed in **bold** are explained in the glossary.

Contents

How many ways can I move?

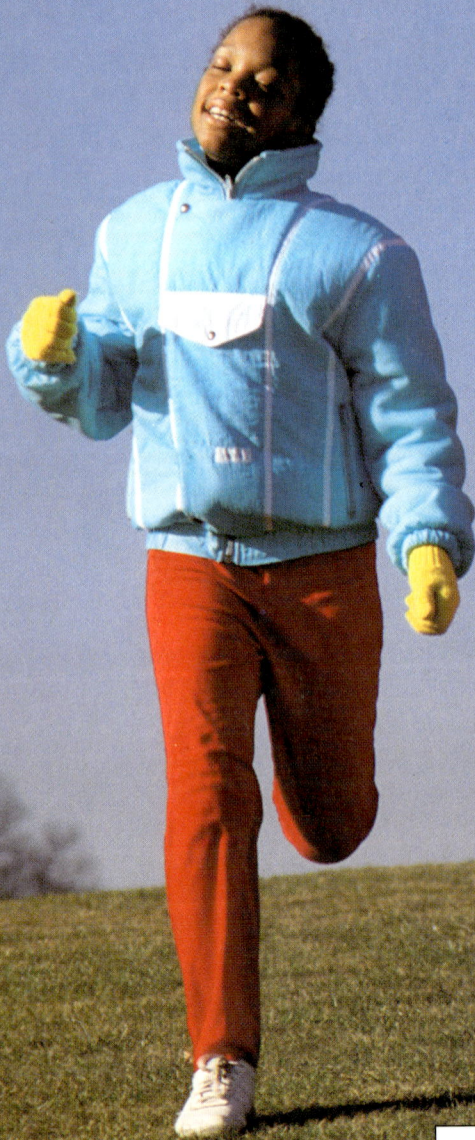

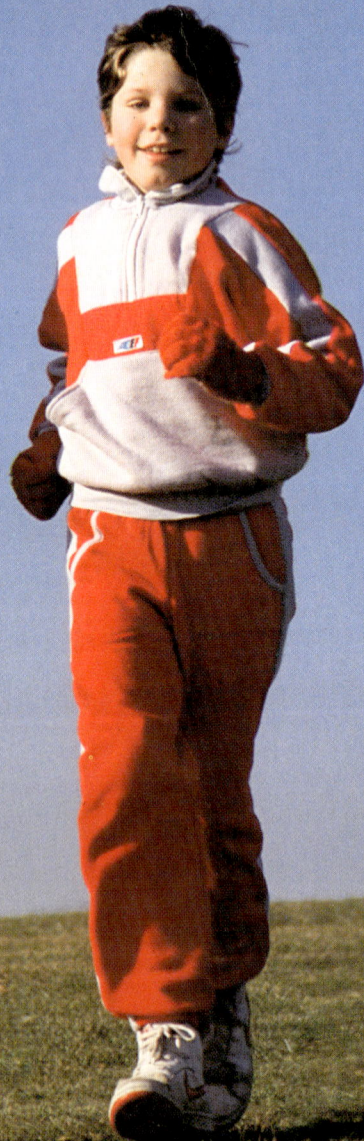

You can run.

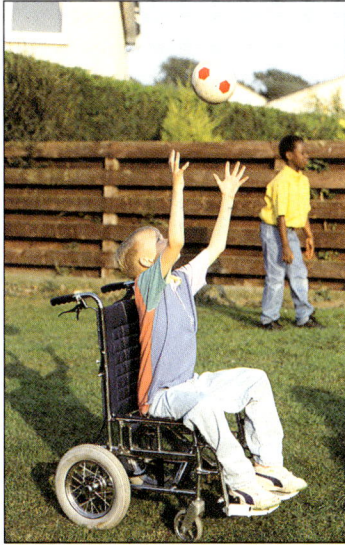

You can throw.

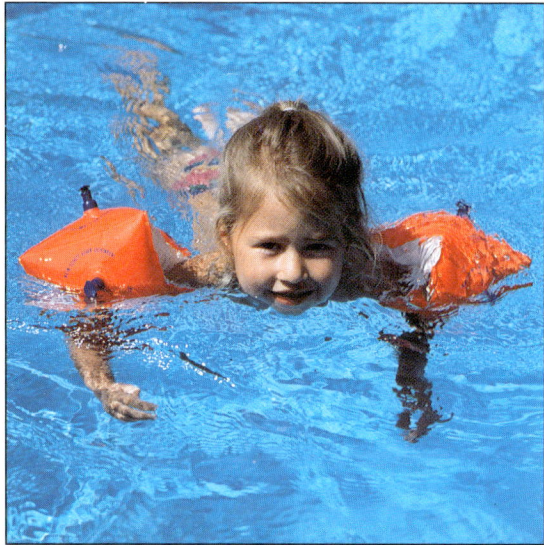

You can swim.

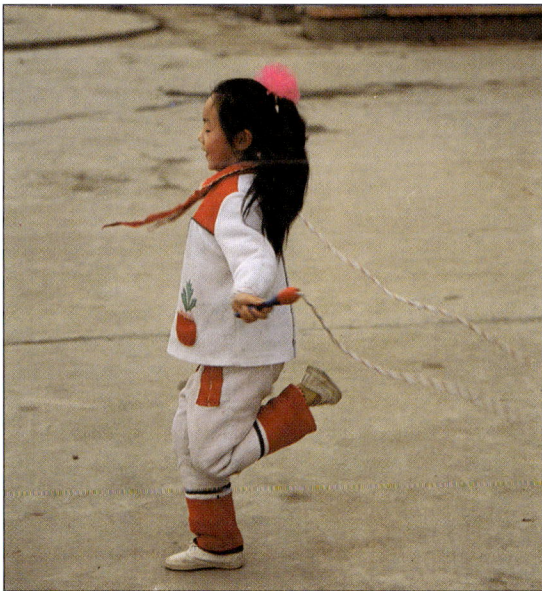

You can skip.

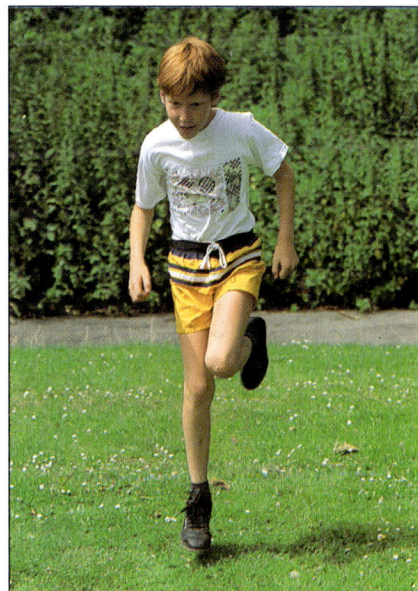

You can hop.

Can you move in any other way?

What makes me move?

This car needs a battery to move. Do you need a battery?

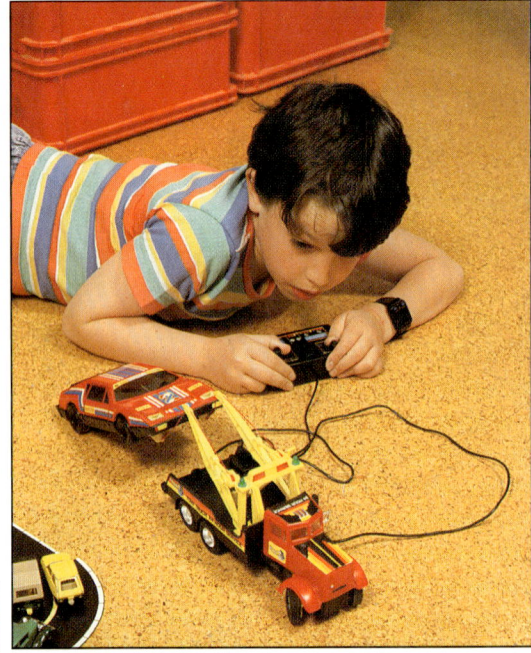

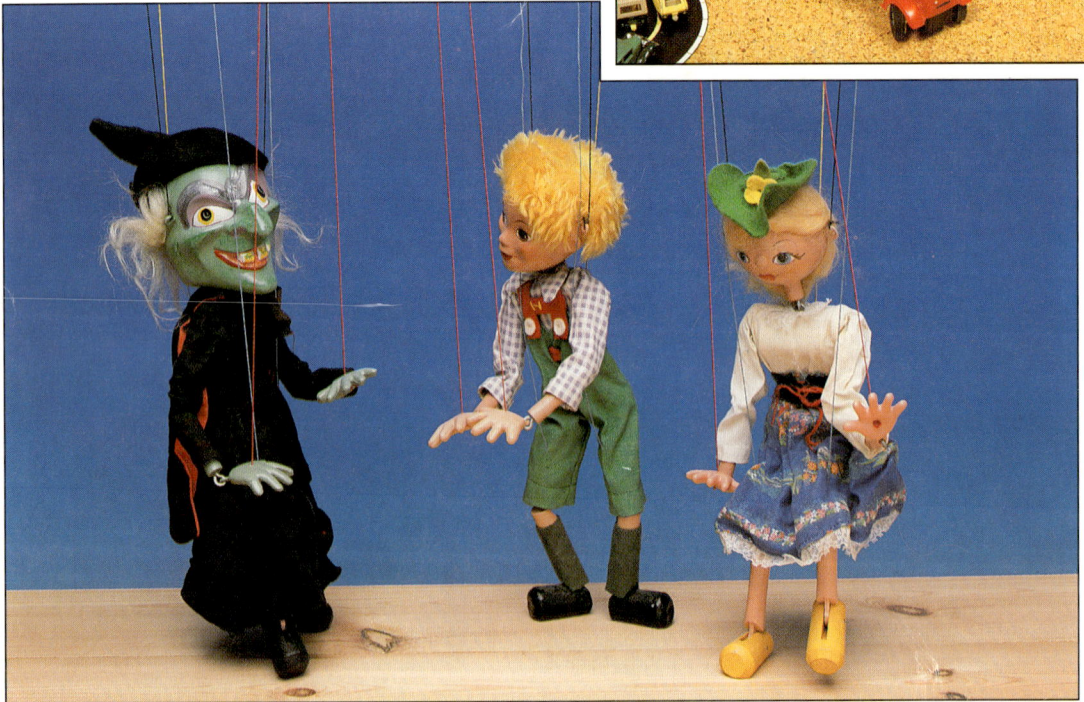

Puppets are moved by strings. Do strings make you move?

These toy frogs spring into the air. Do you have a spring?

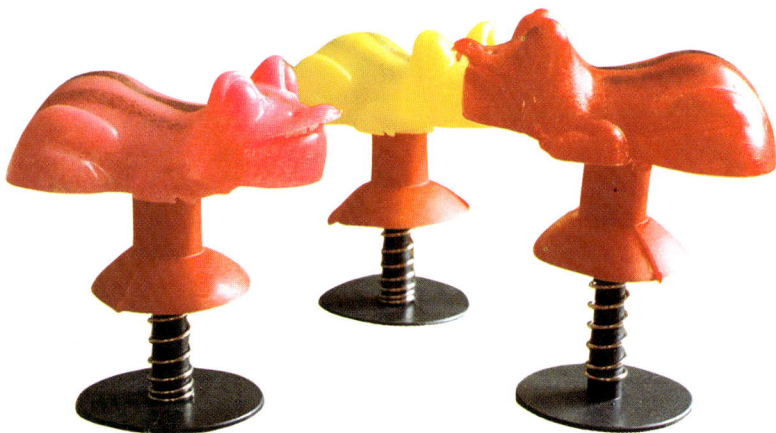

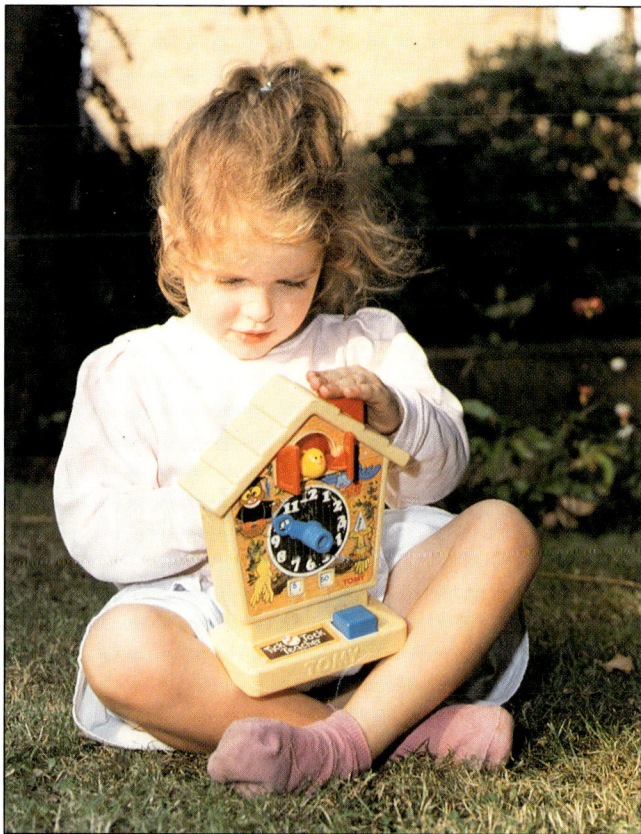

The bird pops out of the clock. It needs a key to wind it up. Do you need a key to make you move?

7

What really makes me move?

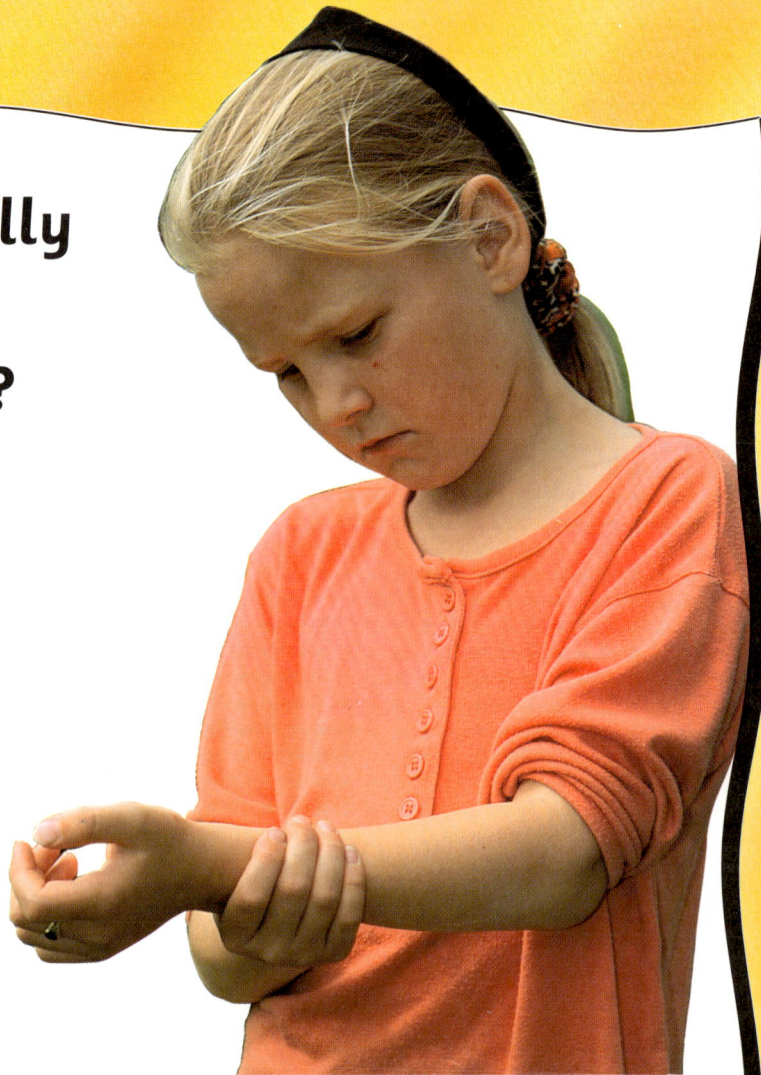

You are not a toy. So you do not use a battery, a spring, a key or strings.

Toys are made of things like plastic, metal, wood or string. What is your body made of?

You cannot see under your skin, but you can feel your **bones** and **muscles**.

How many bones can you feel in your arm? Can you feel any muscles in your arm as well?

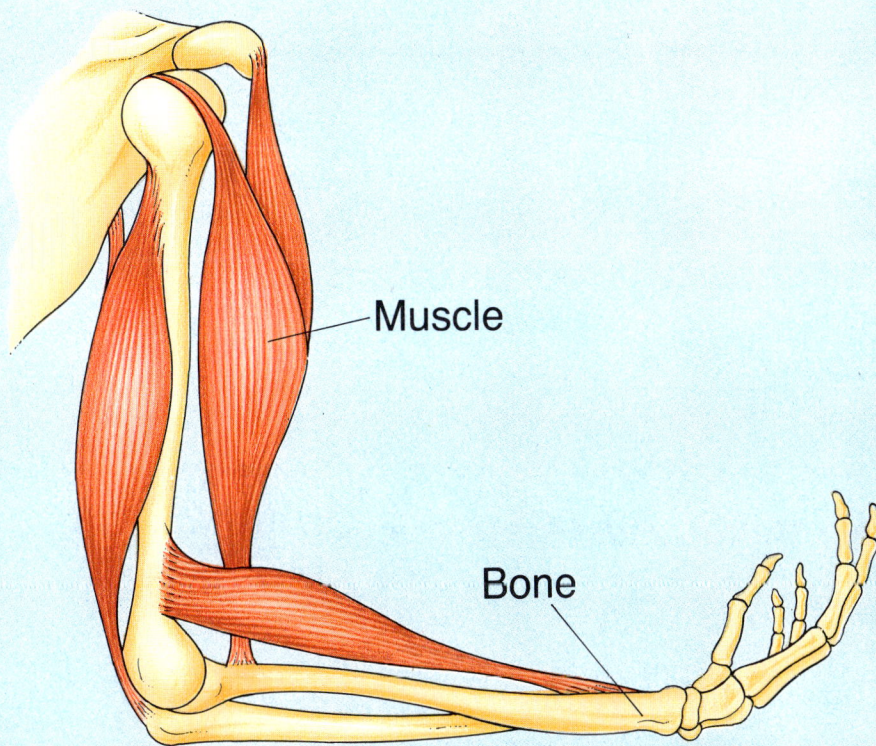

Muscle

Bone

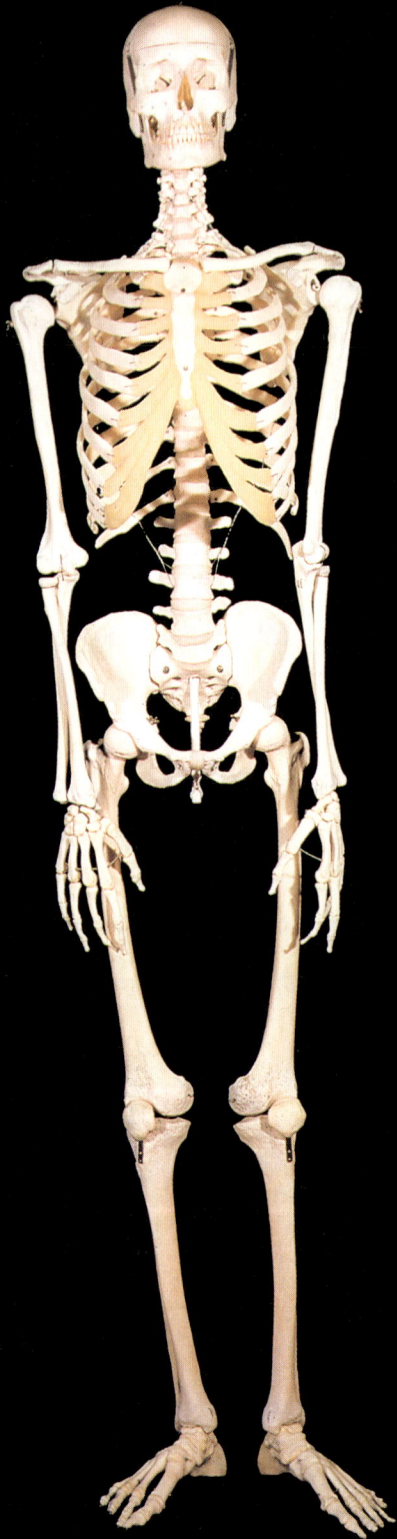

Why do I have a skeleton?

You have 206 bones in your body. All these bones joined together make your **skeleton**. What do you think you would look like without a skeleton?

A skeleton gives you shape and protects parts of your body. What does your skull protect? What do your ribs protect?

The skull and ribs are two parts of the skeleton. Do you know the names of any others? Do you know where they are?

Where would these labels go?

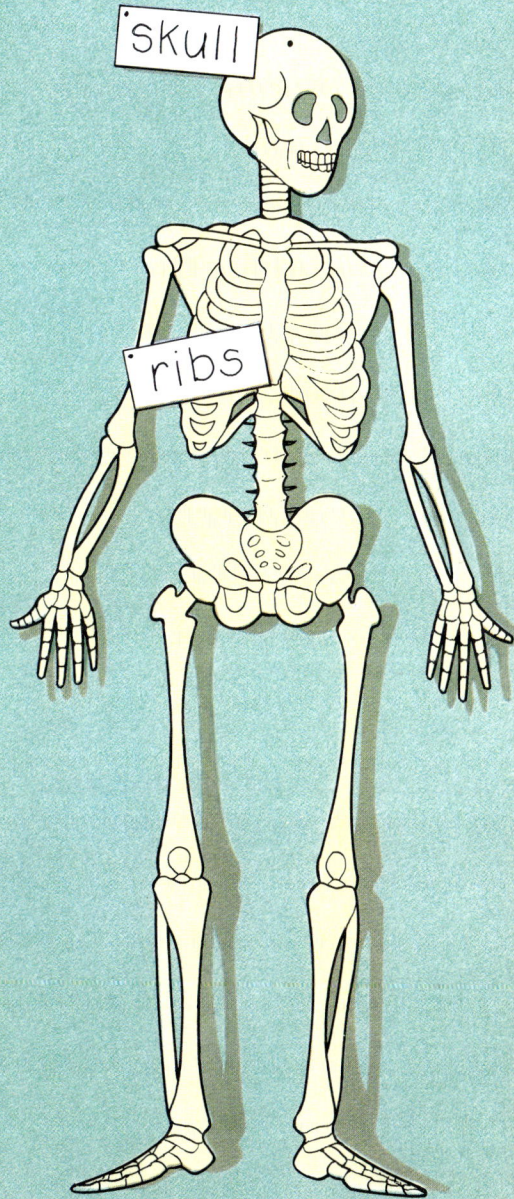

skull

ribs

jaw

thigh

spine

What are bones?

Bones are all different shapes and sizes. This is because they have different jobs to do.

You can feel a curved bone – your **jaw**.

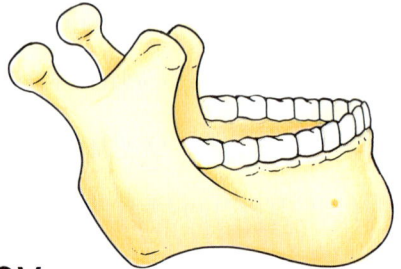

You can feel a bumpy bone – your **spine**.

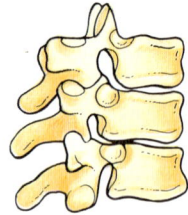

You can feel a long bone – your leg.

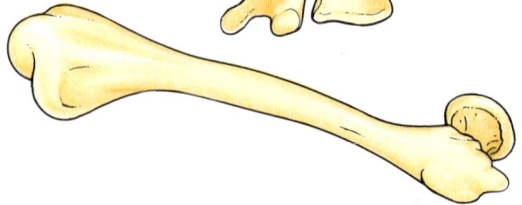

The biggest bone in your body is your **thigh** bone. The smallest bone is in your ear.

For bones to grow strong you need to eat certain foods. Cheese, fresh fruit and green vegetables are good for bones.

You can make a skeleton. You will need card, pencils, scissors and paper fasteners. Copy these bone shapes on to your card and cut them out. Join up your skeleton with paper fasteners.

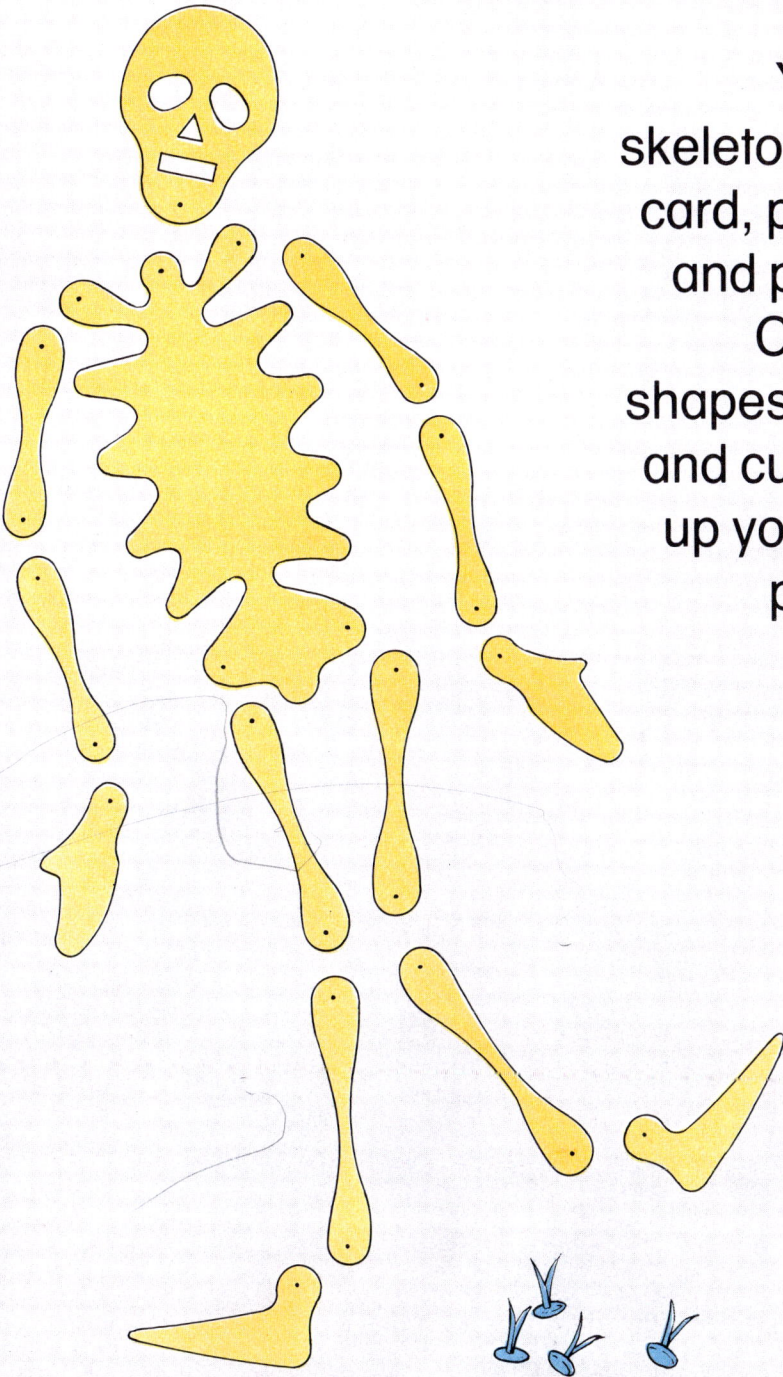

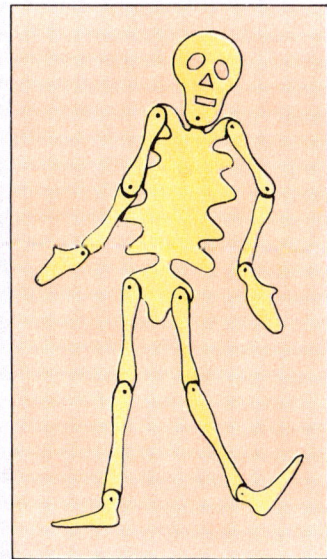

What are muscles?

There are 650 muscles in your body. Without muscles you could not move.

You need muscles to breathe, or to blink. You use muscles when you eat.

Muscles are like bundles of elastic that stretch or bunch up when they are used. This **athlete** has got big muscles.

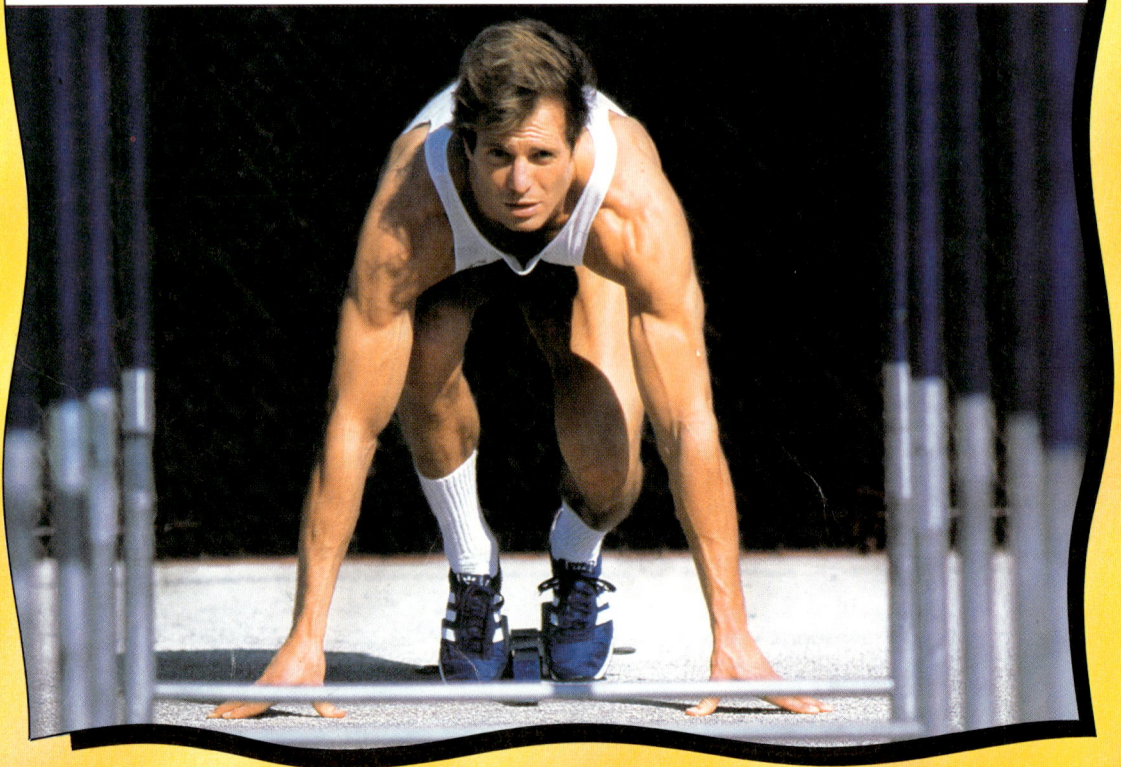

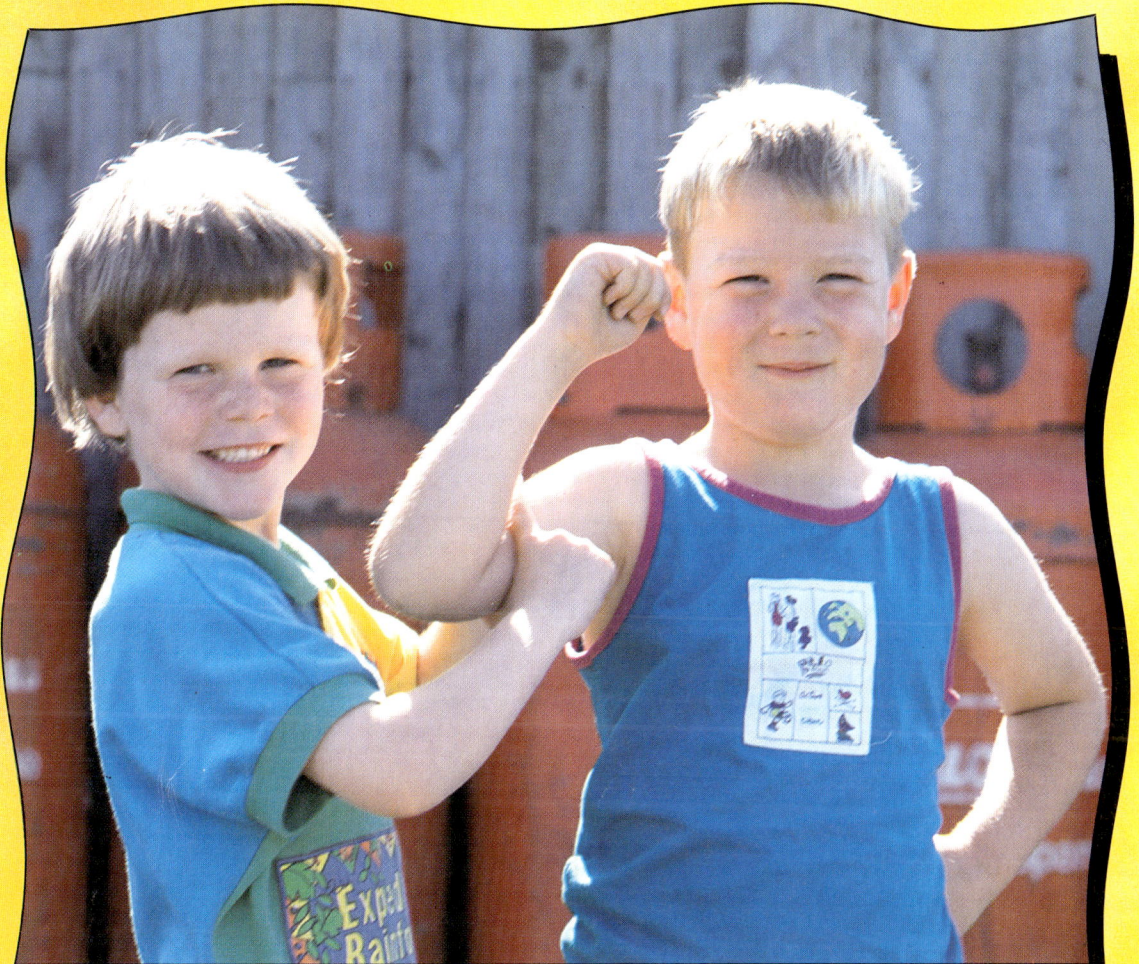

Bend your arm so that your hand touches your shoulder. Can you feel your muscle change shape? This muscle is called the **biceps**.

Can I control my muscles?

You can only control some of your muscles. You can choose to move your arms, legs and other parts of your body. You do not use these muscles all the time, so sometimes they can get tired. Open and close your hand. Count the number of times you can do this before you get tired.

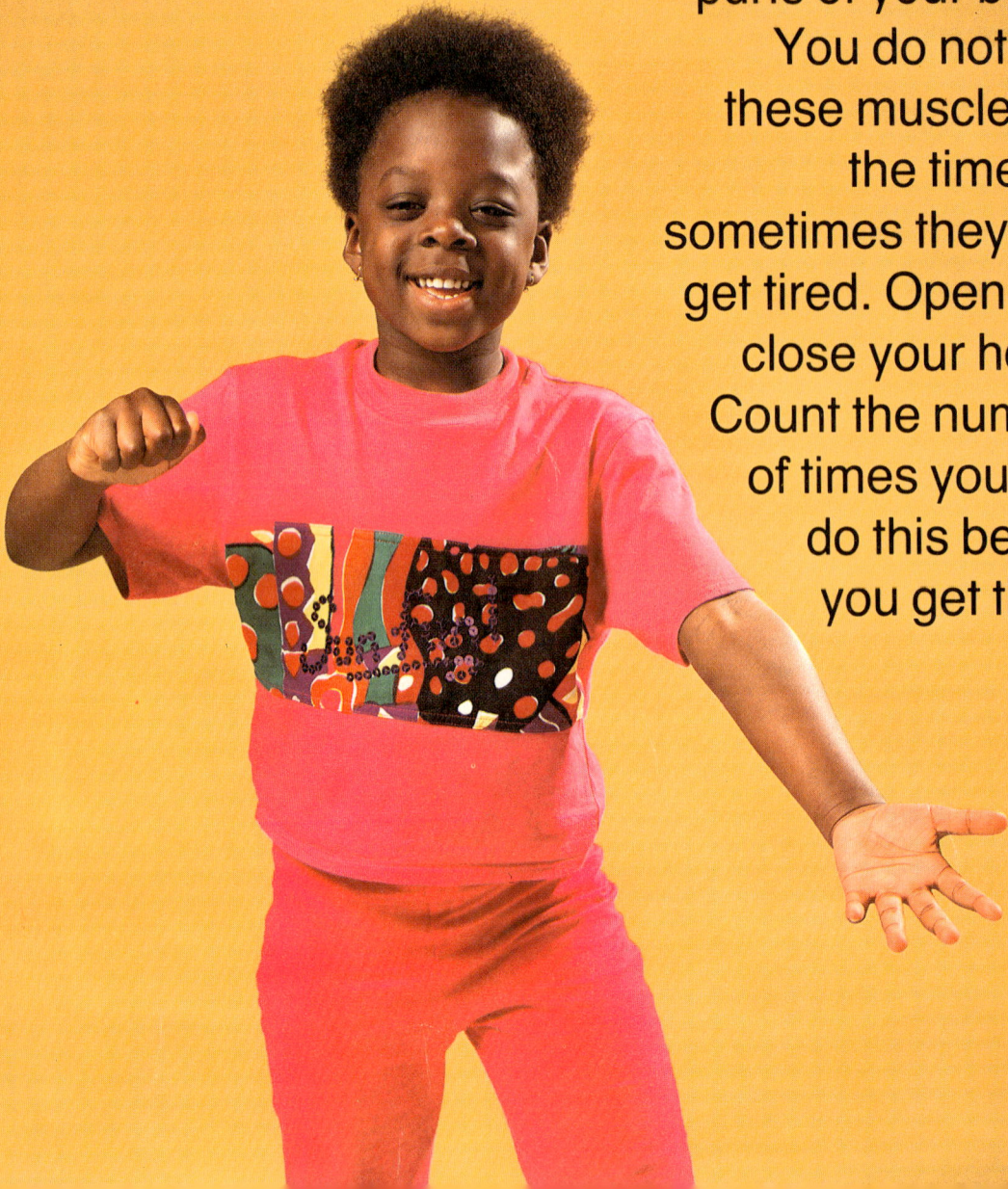

Other muscles work without you thinking about them. Some move your food through your body. Some make you shiver when you are cold. Can you stop yourself shivering?

Your **heart** is a very special muscle. It is working all the time. It moves blood all around your body.

Can you feel your heart working? Does it always feel the same? When does it feel different?

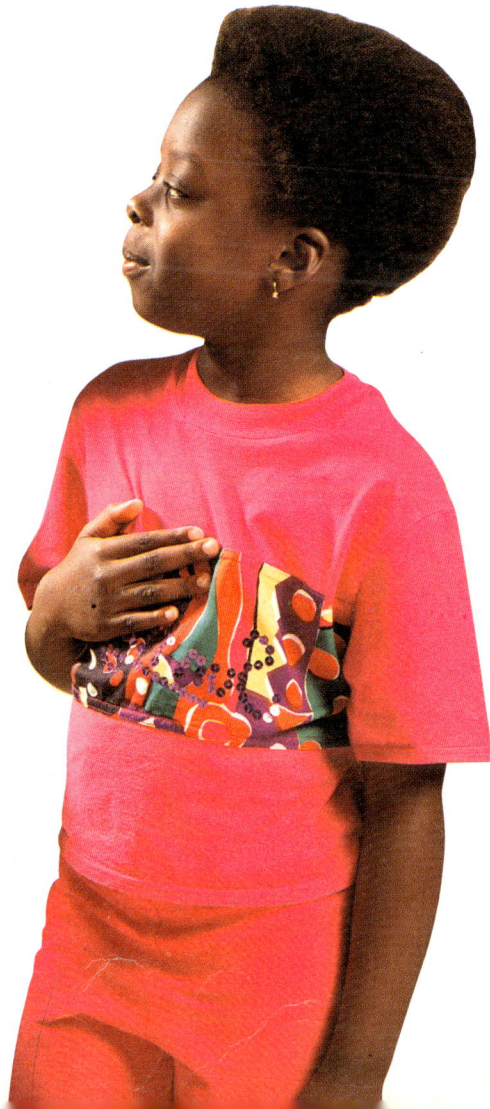

What are they feeling?

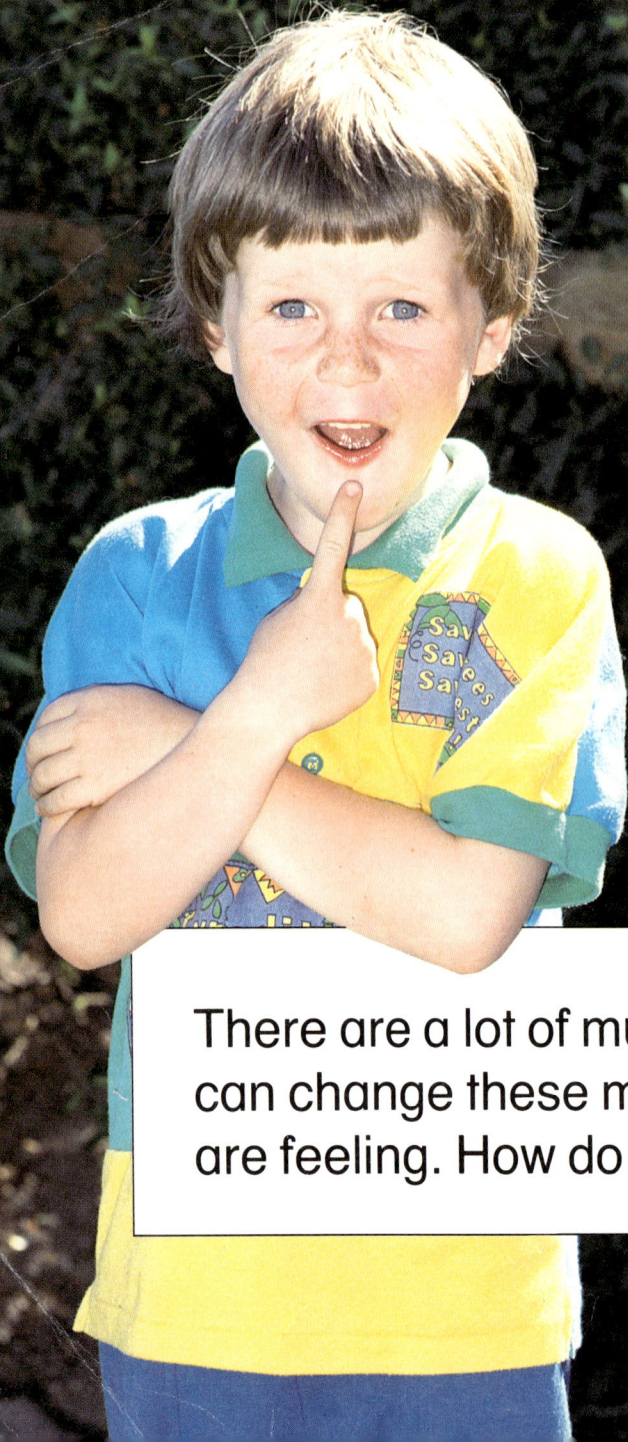

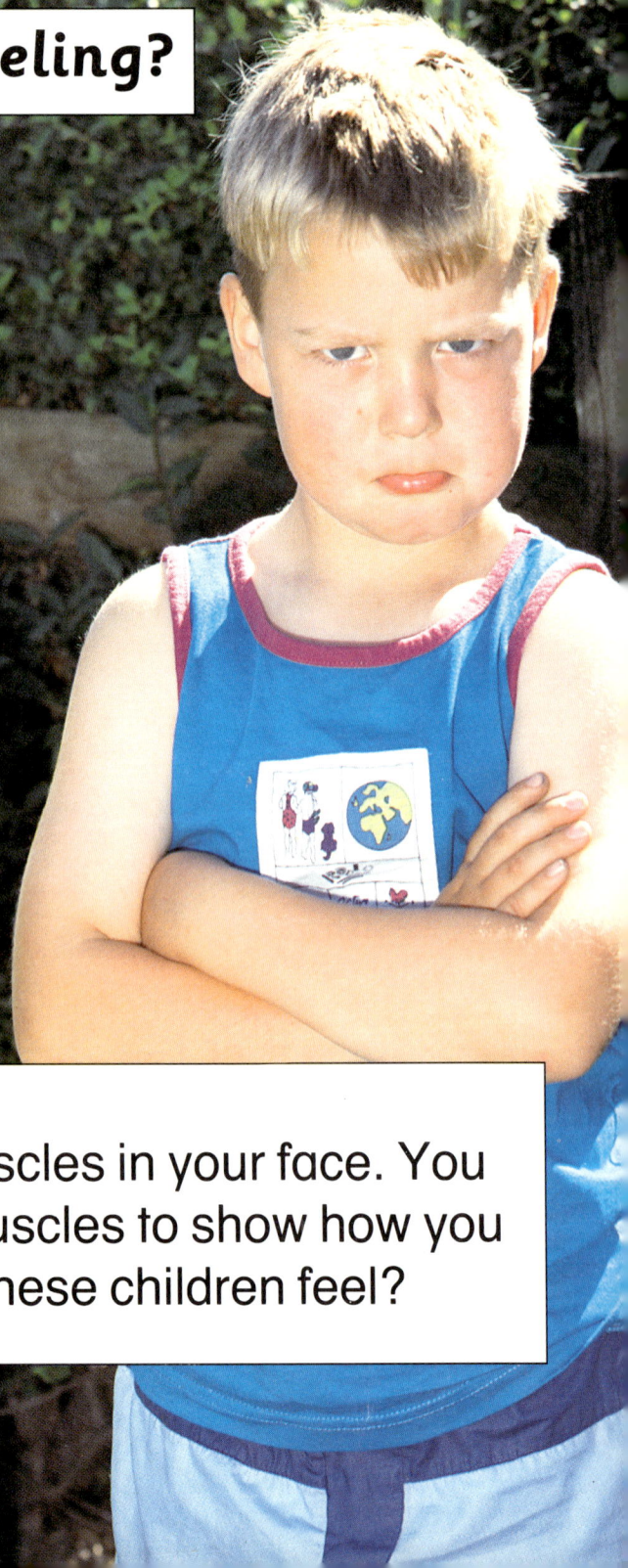

There are a lot of muscles in your face. You can change these muscles to show how you are feeling. How do these children feel?

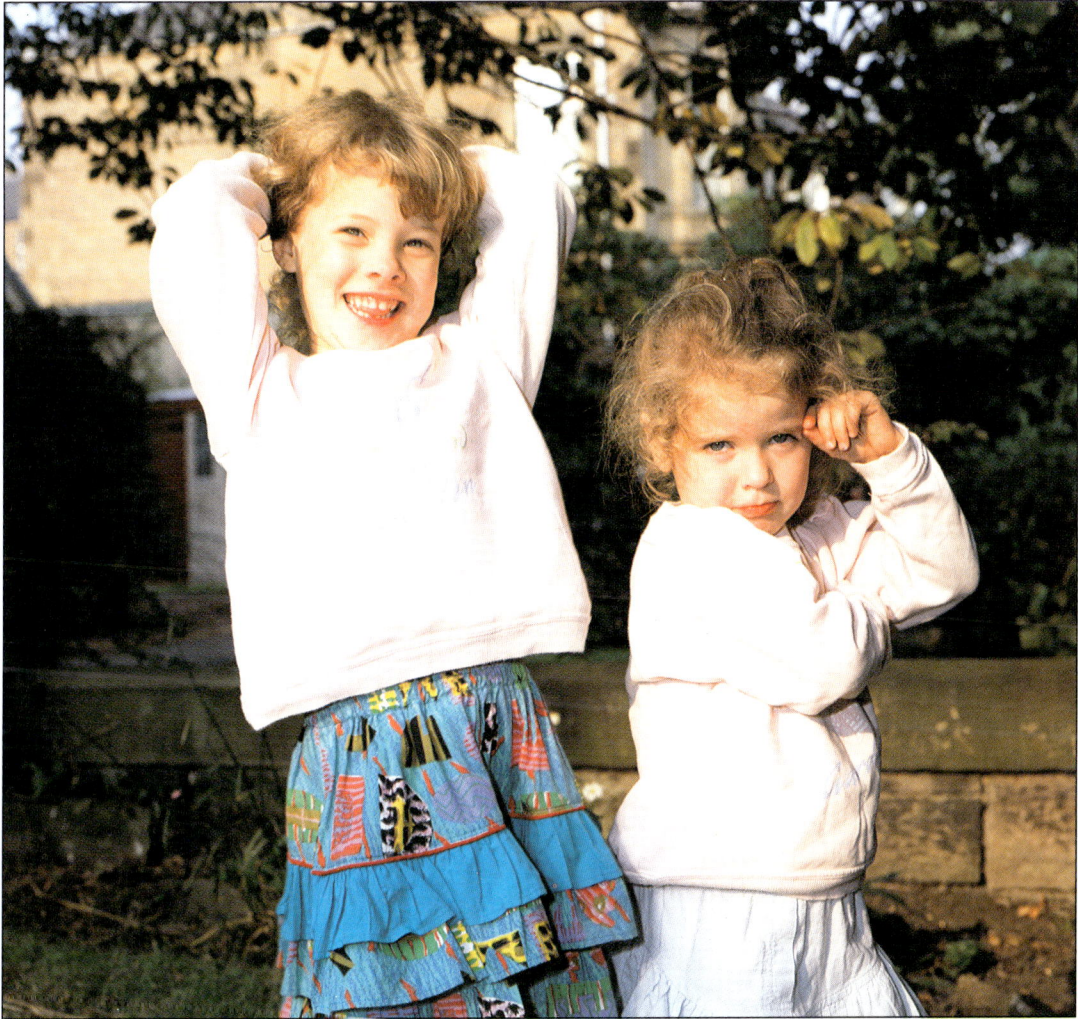

Can you change your face to show what you are feeling?

It is easier to smile than to frown. You only use seventeen muscles when you smile. You use forty muscles when you frown.

What are joints?

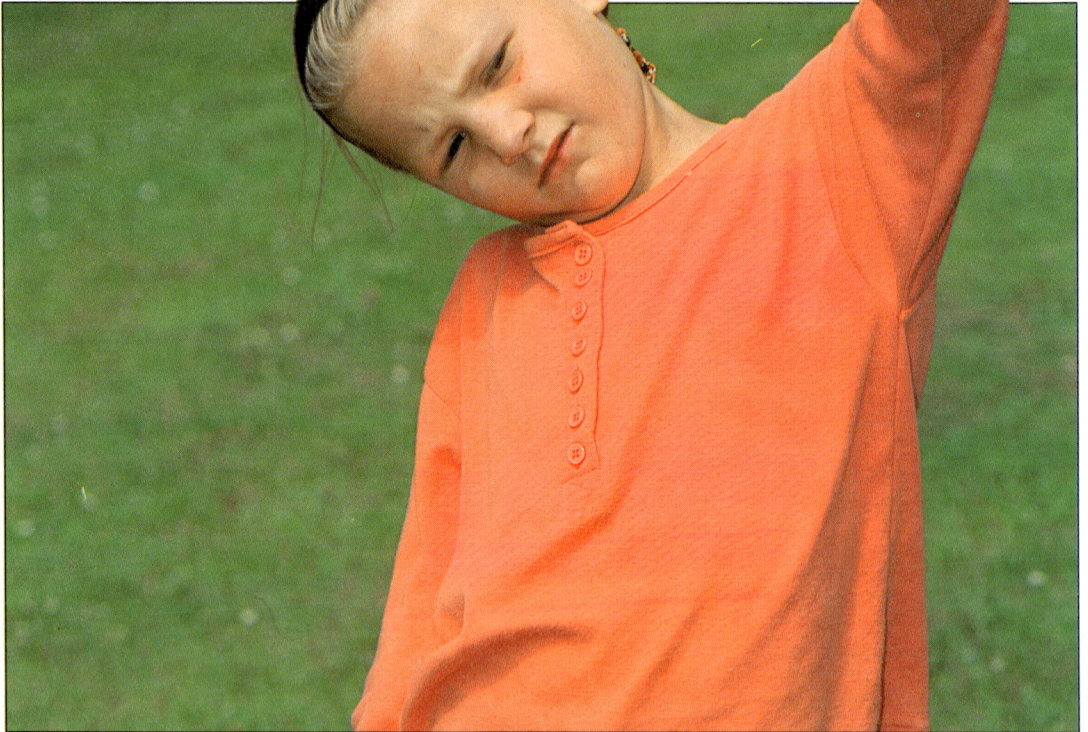

The place where two bones meet is called a **joint**. Bones are joined together in different ways. This helps you move easily.

How does your arm move at the wrist?
How does your arm move at the elbow?
How does your arm move at the shoulder?

How does your head move? Can you think of any other joints in your body?

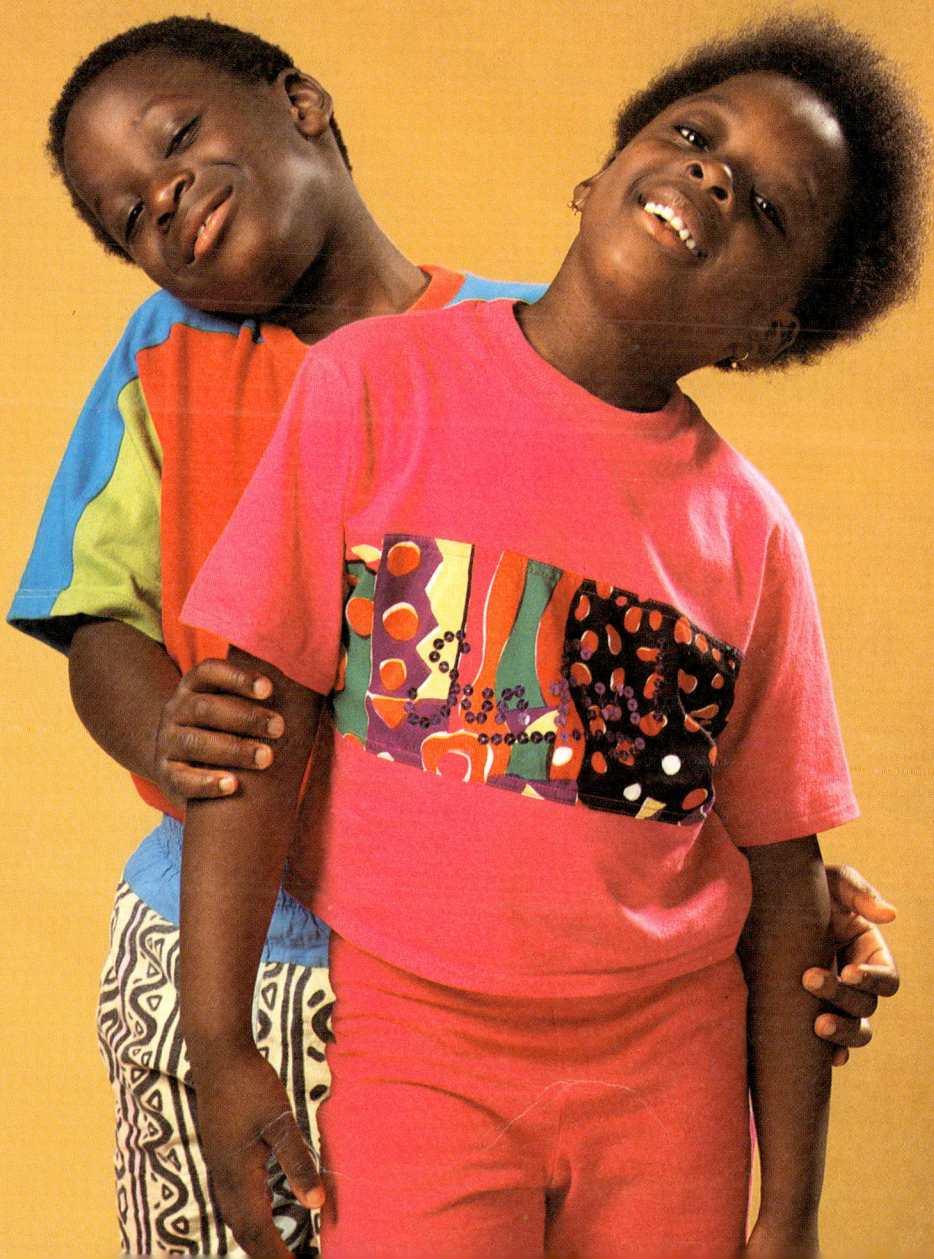

What happens if I break a bone?

Bones are strong and do not break easily. But accidents sometimes happen. Do you know anyone who has broken a bone? How did they do it?

If you break a bone you need to go to hospital for an X-ray. An X-ray is a special photograph which shows the bones inside your body. Look at the broken bone in this X-ray.

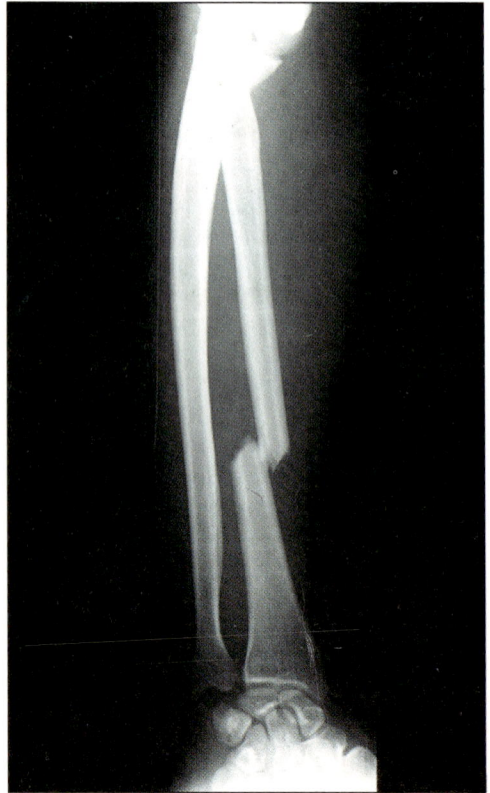

Doctors and nurses at the hospital put the broken bone back together. Then it must be kept still until it has completely mended.

This boy has broken his wrist. He is wearing a **plaster cast** to keep it still.

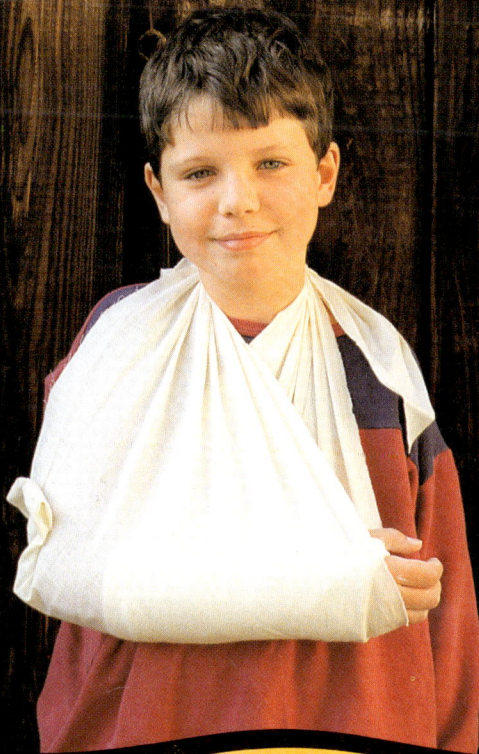

Can we all move easily?

Not everyone can run and skip and play on their own. Some people have difficulty using their muscles or joints. They may need help to move around.

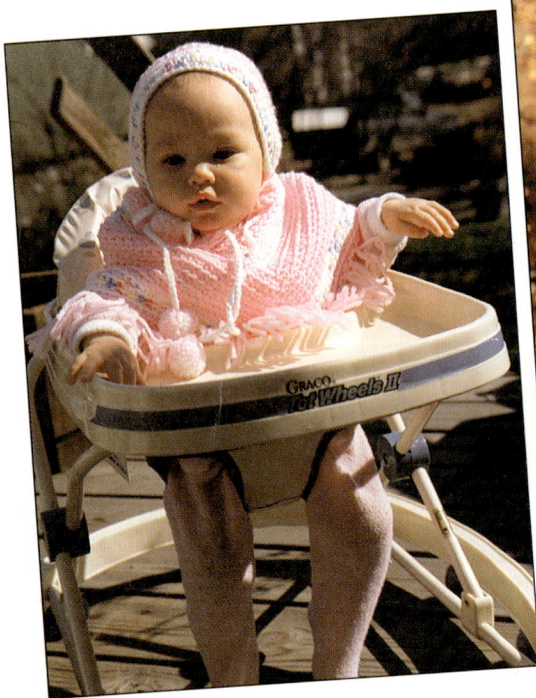

This baby has a baby walker.

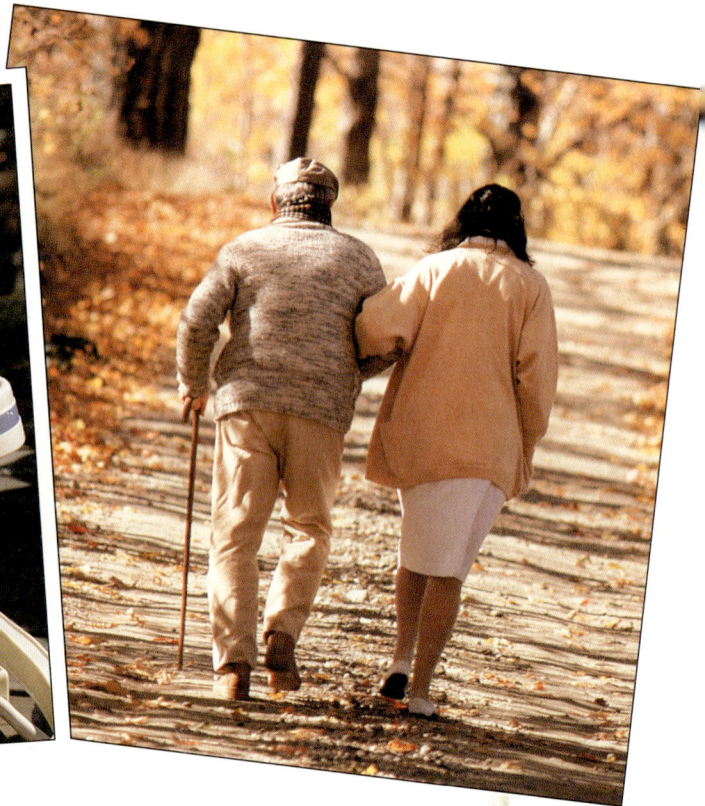

This old man has a stick.

24

Some people need a wheelchair to move around.

This boy can move very quickly in his wheelchair. He is moving as fast as he can to try and win a race.

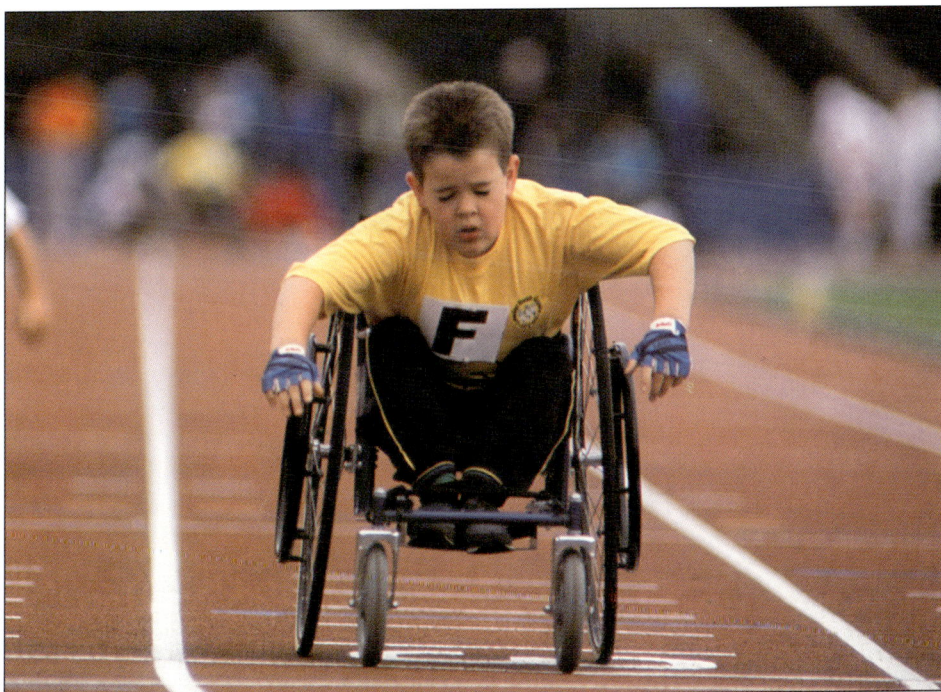

If you were in a wheelchair, what would it be difficult to do? How could some things be made easier?

How do I use my hands?

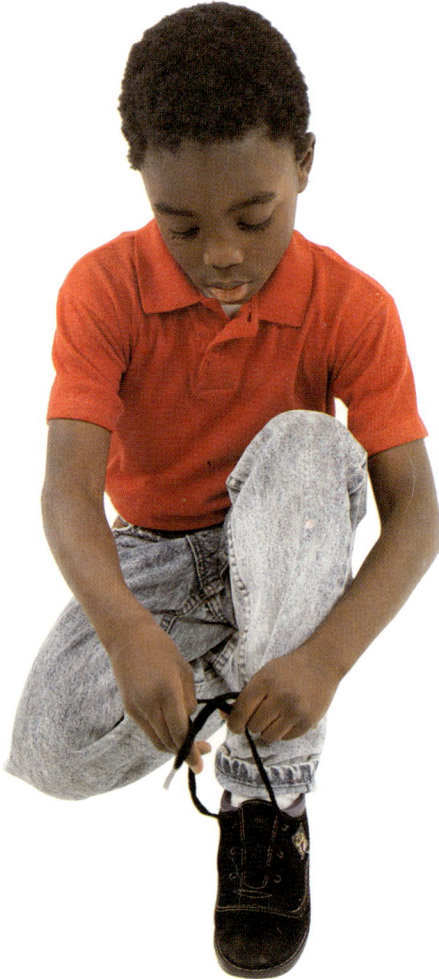

Can you brush
your teeth?

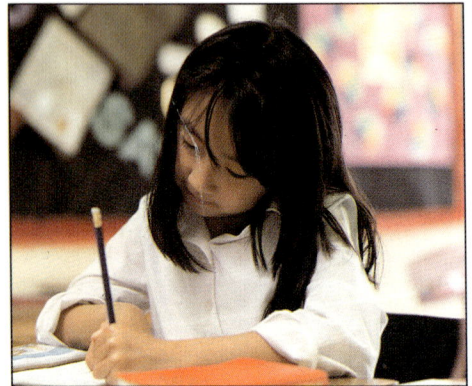

Can you tie
your shoelaces?

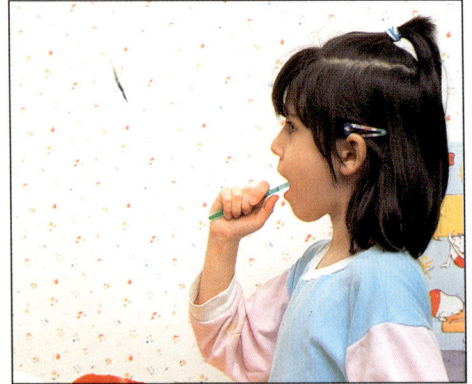

Can you write
your name?

26

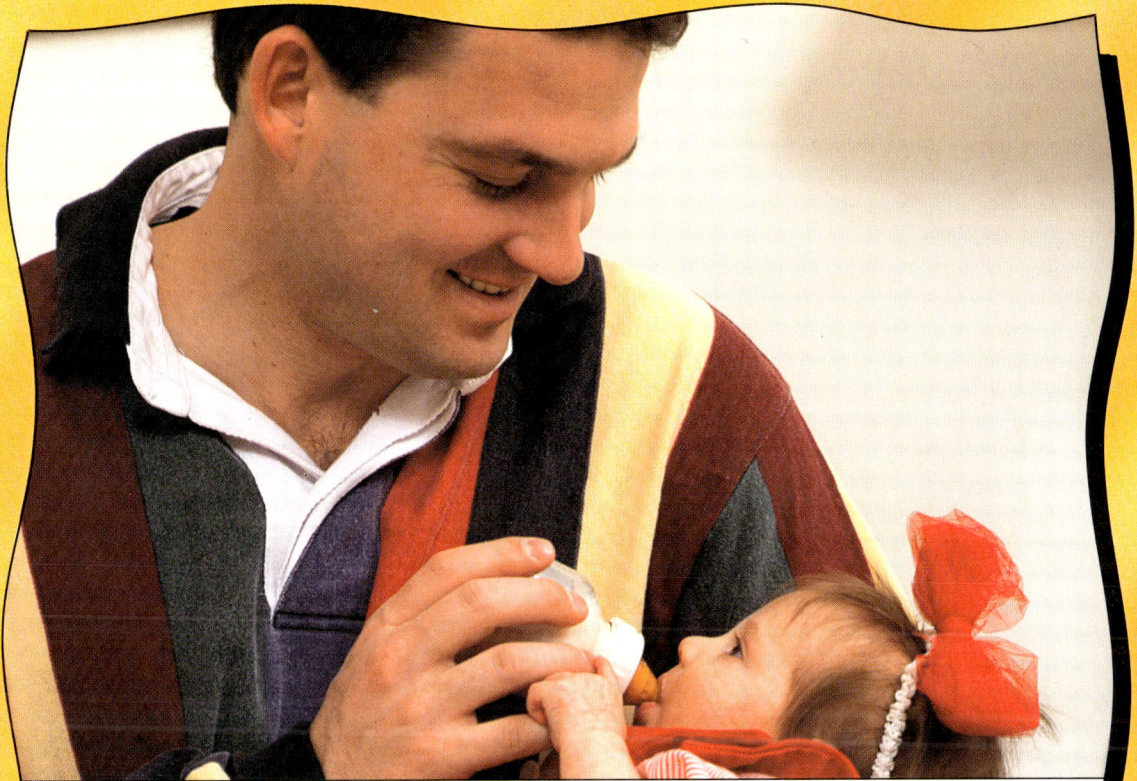

What can you do now that you could not do as a baby?

When you were a baby you needed help to eat, wash and dress. How much help do you need now?

How fast can I move?

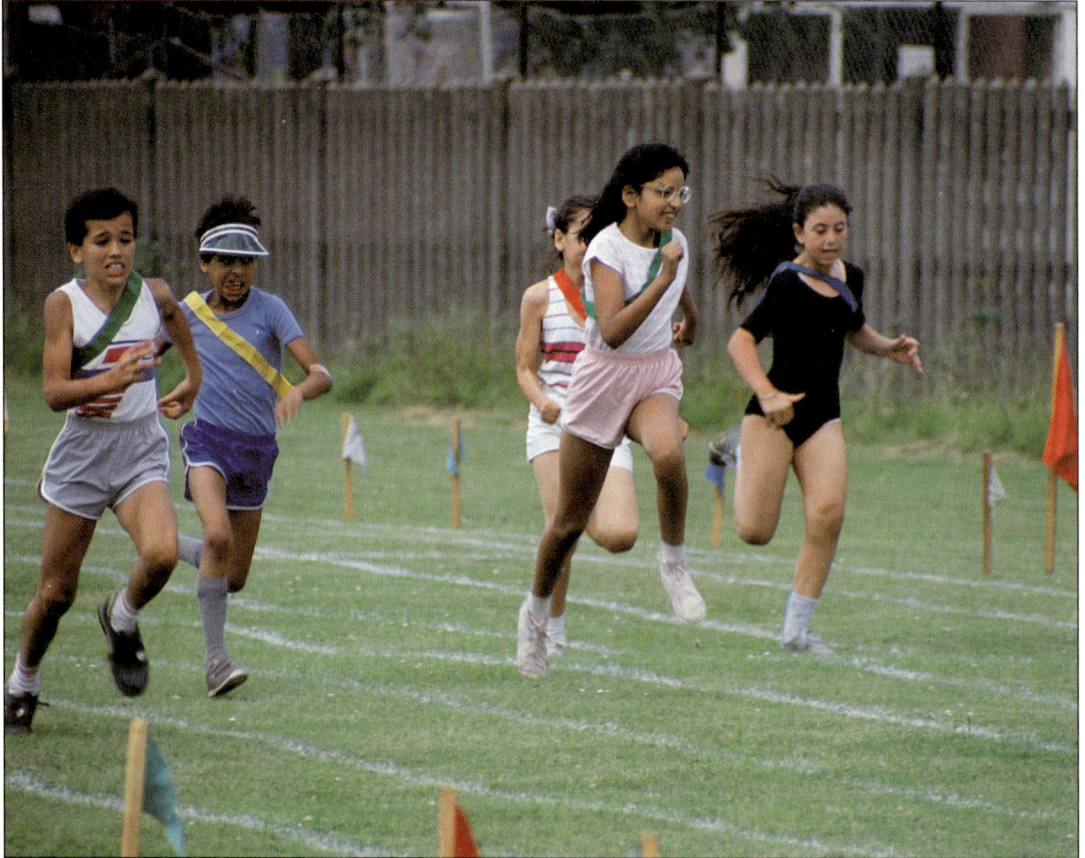

Have you tried to move fast? Some people can move faster than others. They may become athletes.

Athletes use their muscles a lot. This makes the muscles strong.

Exercising your muscles helps you to keep fit and **healthy**. What exercise do you do?

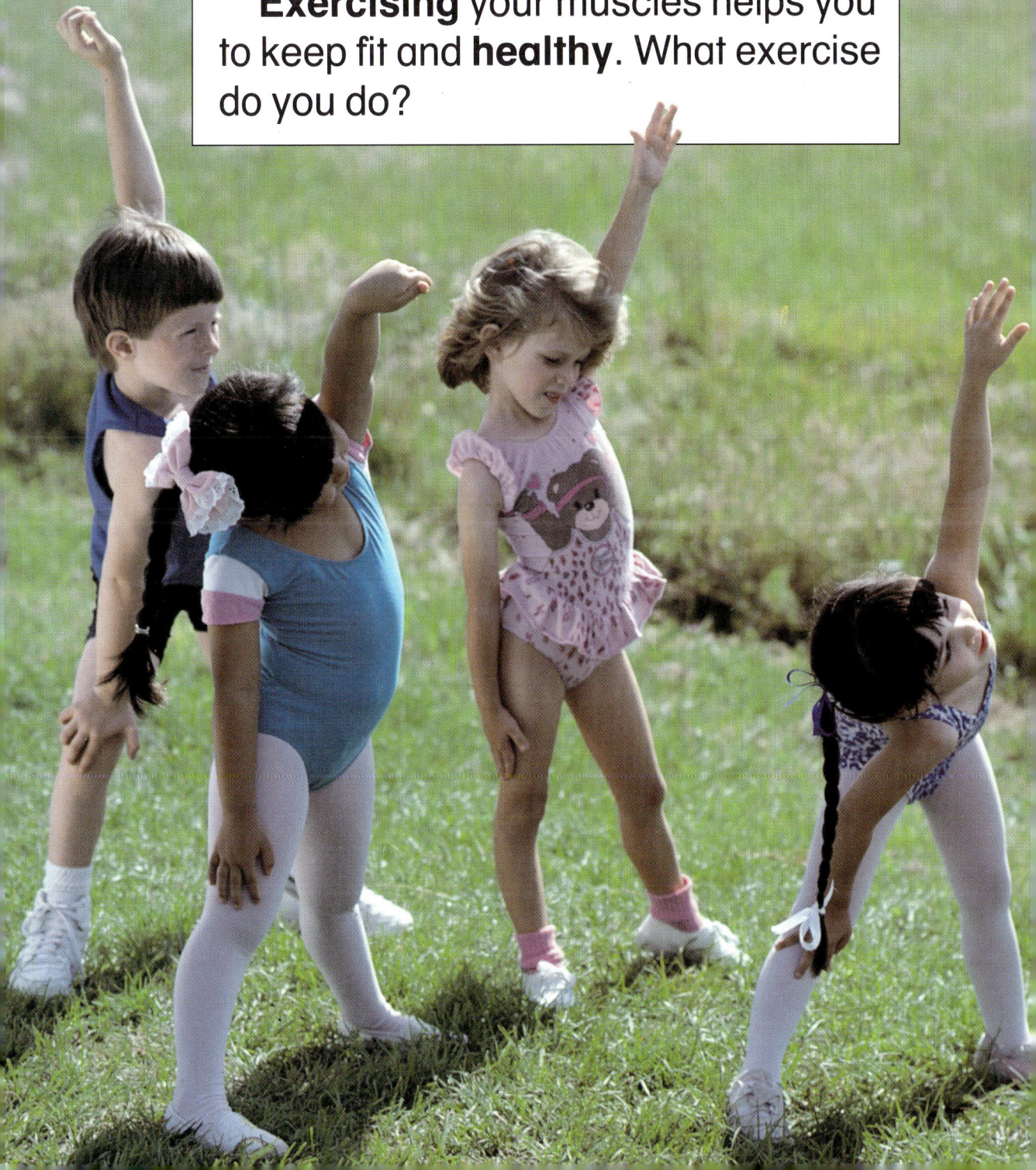

Glossary

Athlete Someone who is good at sports.

Biceps A big muscle in your upper arm.

Bones The hard parts of the body that make up the skeleton.

Exercising Using your muscles a lot, so that they become strong.

Healthy Fit and well.

Heart A muscle that moves blood around the body.

Jaw The chin bone.

Joint A place in your body where two or more bones meet.

Muscles The parts of the body that become tight or loose so that you can move.

Plaster cast A hard casing for mending broken bones.

Skeleton The framework of all the bones in the body.

Spine The backbone.

Thigh The upper part of your leg.

Books to read

Funny Bones by Janet and Allan Ahlberg (Heinemann, 1982)

How My Body Works by Althea (Dinosaur, 1989)

Feelings by Aliki Brandenberg (Pan Books, 1989)

Avocado Baby by John Burningham (Collins, 1986)

Moving by Joy Richardson (Hodder & Stoughton, 1991)

Notes on the National Curriculum

This book is relevant to the following Attainment Targets:

	Level	Statements of Attainment
SCIENCE (Draft Orders October 1991) Attainment Target 1: Scientific investigation	1	*Pupils should:* carry out investigations in which they: (a) observe familiar materials and events.
	2	carry out investigations in which they: (a) ask questions such as 'how . . . ?', 'why . . . ?' and 'what will happen if . . . ?', suggest ideas and make predictions. (b) make a series of related observations.
Attainment Target 2: Life and living processes	1	(a) be able to name the external parts of the human body and the flowering plant. (b) know that there is a wide variety of living things which includes humans.
	3	(a) know the basic life processes common to humans and other animals.
Attainment Target 4: Physical processes	1	(a) understand that things can be moved by pushing or pulling them.
	2	(d) understand that pushes and pulls can make things start moving, speed up, slow down or stop.
MATHEMATICS Attainment Target 1:	1	*Pupils should:* (c) make predictions based on experience.
	2	(c) respond appropriately to the question 'What would happen if . . . ?'
Attainment Target 2:	1	(a) use number in the context of classroom and school.
ENGLISH		Children using this book can cover many aspects of the *Reading, Speaking* and *Listening* sections of the English National Curriculum.

Index

Picture acknowledgements
The publishers would like to thank the following: Chapel Studios 6 bottom, 7 top, 26 left, 26 top right; Eye Ubiquitous 5 bottom left (J. Waterlow), 5 bottom right (Y. Nikiteas), 8 (Y. Nikiteas), 20 (Y. Nikiteas), 25 (P. Blake); PHOTRI 24 left; Science Photo Library 10 (M. Kaye), 22 (J. Stevenson); Tony Stone Worldwide 14 (P. Langone); Wayland Picture Library (A. Blackburn) 5 top left, 7 bottom, 15, 16, 17, 18, 19, 21; Timothy Woodcock 4, 6 top, 23, 28; Zefa 5 top right (Mueller), 24 right, 26 bottom right, 27, 30. Artwork on pages 9, 11, 12 and 13 supplied by John Yates. Background artwork on pages 8-9, 14-15, 22-3 and 26-7 supplied by Jenny Hughes.